FATTY LIVER DIET COOKBOOK

Your Definitive Guide with Easy, Delicious, and Quick Recipes to Heal Your Liver and Feel Great Fast | Includes a Step-by-Step Action Plan and Scientifically Proven Advice

Dr. Maggie A. White

Limited Liability

Please note that the content of this book is based on personal experience and various information sources, and it is only for personal use.

Please note the information contained within this document is for educational and entertainment purposes only and no warranties of any kind are declared or implied.

Readers acknowledge that the author is not engaged in providing medical, dietary, nutritional or professional advice, or physical training. Please consult a doctor, nutritionist or dietician, before attempting any techniques outlined in this book.

Nothing in this book is intended to replace common sense or medical consultation or professional advice and is meant only to inform.

Your particular circumstances may not be suited to the example illustrated in this book; in fact, they likely will not be. You should use the information in this book at your own risk. The reader is responsible for his or her actions.

The information provided herein is stated to be truthful and consistent, in that any liability, in terms of inattention or otherwise, by any usage or abuse of any policies, processes, or directions contained within is the solitary and utter responsibility of the recipient reader.

By reading this book, the reader agrees that under no circumstances is the author responsible for any losses, direct or indirect, which are incurred as a result of the use of the information contained within this document, including, but not limited to, errors, omissions, or inaccuracies.

CONTENTS

PART

1

WHAT IS FATTY LIVER DISEASE?

Fatty Liver Disease

Fatty liver disease, also referred to as hepatic steatosis, is a medical condition characterized by the accumulation of fat within the liver cells. This buildup of fat can damage the liver, potentially leading to cirrhosis, a serious condition characterized by permanent scarring and liver damage. Cirrhosis can further progress to liver cancer or liver failure. However, you can manage and slow the progression of fatty liver by opting for a healthier diet and incorporating regular physical activity into your routine.

In addition to choosing a low-carb eating style, the manner in which food is cooked is also important to optimize the diet's results.

Approximately **30%** of adults in the U.S. have non-alcoholic fatty liver disease (NAFLD). Most individuals are unaware they have NAFLD, as signs and symptoms typically do not manifest until significant and irreversible damage, such as cirrhosis, has occurred.

NAFLD heightens the risk of developing cardiovascular disease, which is the leading cause of death among those with NAFLD. Cardiovascular disease further raises the likelihood of experiencing a heart attack or heart failure.

HOW FATTY LIVER DISEASE DEVELOPS

The primary cause of NAFLD is being overweight.

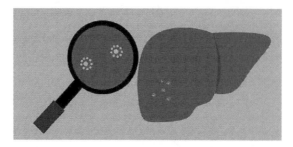

The adipose tissue within our bodies consistently releases fatty acids into the bloodstream, subsequently making their way to the liver..

In addition to being overweight, consuming a diet rich in sweets, starchy foods, and processed snacks contributes to the development of NAFLD. These foods are known as simple carbohydrates.

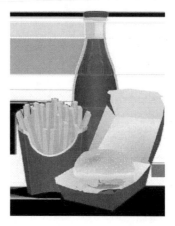

Simple carbohydrates are converted into fat by the liver and are also stored in our bodies as fat deposits.

As time passes, the liver becomes burdened by the surplus of fat from both the bloodstream and dietary intake. Consequently, the liver begins to store fat within its cells, leading to its enlargement

With the accumulation of fat in the liver, inflammation gradually develops. This inflammation can initiate a process of permanent scarring in the liver cells, known as fibrosis. Over time, this scarring can progress to a more severe condition called cirrhosis, wherein the liver becomes extensively scarred and its function deteriorates. Eventually, cirrhosis may lead to liver failure, necessitating a liver transplant for survival.

Once inflammation sets in within the liver, the process of scarring commences. Non-alcoholic steatohepatitis (NASH) refers to the inflammatory state within the liver. When cirrhosis arises, the liver's capacity to heal and operate efficiently diminishes. Cirrhosis heightens the likelihood of liver cancer and could necessitate a liver transplant if liver function significantly declines.

NAFLD may arise if you:

- ➢ Are overweight or obese
- ➢ Have prediabetes or Type II diabetes
- ➢ Experience high blood pressure
- ➢ Have elevated cholesterol levels

DIAGNOSIS OF NAFLD

NAFLD can be identified through ultrasound imaging and blood tests. Your physician might suggest a liver biopsy to gauge the severity of your liver condition and tailor a treatment strategy accordingly.

TREATING NAFLD

Treatment for NAFLD primarily involves:

- ➢ Aiming for a 5–10% reduction in body weight, which is optimal for reversing NAFLD effects. However, dietary modifications alone can yield positive outcomes for the liver.
- ➢ Avoiding alcohol is essential to prevent worsening liver damage.
- ➢ Adopting specific dietary modifications
- ➢ Maintaining a regular exercise routine.

Additionally, depending on the findings of your liver biopsy, your doctor may prescribe medications to assist in treating NAFLD.

PART

2

DIETARY CONSIDERATIONS & FOOD CATEGORIES

THE BASICS

1 Strive to prioritize water, unsweetened tea, or coffee as your main beverages. Steer clear of sugary drinks such as soda, fruit juice, lemonade, and sports drinks.

2 Ensure that half of your plate consists of fruits and vegetables, with an emphasis on non-starchy vegetables and whole fruits.

3 Opt for leaner protein sources like fish, poultry, beans, and nuts, while minimizing intake of red meats, deli meats, bacon, and other processed meats.

4 Choose whole grains such as brown rice, oatmeal, or whole wheat pasta, while paying attention to portion sizes.

5 Utilize olive or canola oil for cooking and in salads, while restricting the use of butter and avoiding trans fats.

6 Engage in physical activity for at least 30 minutes each day. Whether it's taking a brisk walk, doing yard work, or dancing, any activity that gets your heart rate up is beneficial.

FRUITS AND VEGETABLES: WHY ARE THEY IMPORTANT?

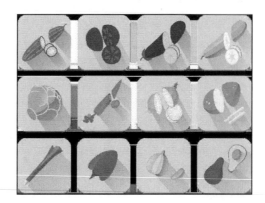

Fruits and vegetables provide carbohydrates primarily from fiber, which helps protect your liver, heart, and digestive system. Fiber-rich foods help you feel full longer and are also packed with antioxidants that may reduce inflammation in your body.

Consuming a diet rich in fruits and vegetables can assist in weight loss and in lowering cholesterol and blood pressure. Initially, you might experience gas or bloating if you're not used to high-fiber foods, but this will subside as your body adjusts.

Starch is another type of carbohydrate known as a "simple carbohydrate." Easily digestible carbohydrates such as starch can rapidly elevate blood sugar levels and might be transformed into fat upon reaching the liver.

Fruits and vegetables can be categorized as "starchy" or "non-starchy," with non-starchy vegetables generally being the healthier choice. A diet abundant in fruits and vegetables can help manage and control NAFLD, aid in weight loss, and prevent or manage type II diabetes.

ABOUT VEGETABLES

- ➢ Aim to consume 4-5 servings of vegetables daily, focusing on non-starchy varieties.
- ➢ Consume vegetables in various preparations, such as raw, roasted, sautéed, grilled, blanched, or in soups.
- ➢ Refrain from combining starches and grains; if you include a starchy vegetable, omit grains from that meal.
- ➢ Avoid fried foods, including fried vegetables like French fries and potato chips..

Examples of Non-Starchy Vegetables	Examples of Starchy Vegetables
Artichoke	Beans (black, kidney, navy, pinto)
Asparagus	Butternut Squash
Baby Corn	Cassava
Bell Peppers	Chickpeas
Beets	Corn
Brussels Sprouts	Lentils
Broccoli/ Cabbage/ Cauliflower	Peas
Carrots	Vegetable Juices
Celery	Yams
Chayote	Sweet Potatoes
Cucumber	White Potatoes
Eggplant	
Leeks	
Okra	
Radishes	

Salad Greens	
Spinach	
Turnips	
Tomato	
Zucchini	

ABOUT FRUIT

➤ Aim to eat 2-3 servings of fruit daily. However, it's crucial to avoid excessive fruit intake.

➤ Choose whole fruits, as they are rich in fiber and natural sugars, which are healthier carbohydrates.

➤ Restrict the consumption of dried fruits, as they frequently contain added sugars detrimental to liver health.

➤ Opt for canned or frozen fruits without added sugars or those packed in 100% fruit juice.

➤ Steer clear of fruit juices. They often contain added sugars, lack the beneficial fiber found in whole fruits, and are easy to overconsume.

FRUITS TO EAT MORE OF	
Fruit	Examples
Berries	Blueberries, Cranberries, Raspberries, Strawberries
Melons	Cantaloupe, Honeydew, Watermelon
Stone Fruits	Cherries, Peaches, Plums
Citrus	Oranges
Others	Grapes

ABOUT GRAINS

Some grains are "complex carbohydrates," while others are "simple carbohydrates." Complex carbohydrates are more beneficial for your well-being.

Guidelines

Limit grain intake to 3-4 servings per day,	Excessive consumption can contribute to weight gain and exacerbate NAFLD.
Opt for whole grain products	They provide complex carbohydrates, promoting prolonged satiety and energy levels..
Avoid combining starchy vegetables with grains	If eating a starchy vegetable, skip grains for that meal.
Enhance your grains with vegetables	Add vegetables to dishes like rice or pasta to increase fiber.

Grains to Embrace (Complex Carbohydrates)	Grains to Moderate (Simple Carbohydrates)
100% whole grain or whole wheat bread products	Instant oatmeal
Quinoa Whole grain or multi-grain crackers	White pasta
Corn tortillas	White bread products (muffins, bread, bagels)
Not instant Oatmeal	White rice
Brown or wild rice	
Whole wheat flour tortillas	
Quinoa	
Whole wheat flour (for baking)	
Air-popped popcorn	
Whole wheat pasta	

WHAT ARE SIMPLE CARBOHYDRATES?

➢ Simple carbohydrates, also known as processed foods, lack nutritional value and contribute to NAFLD and weight gain.

➢ Snack items, candies, desserts, and sweetened beverages fall under the category of simple carbohydrates.

➢ Simple carbohydrates are often labeled as "added sugar," so it's essential to check nutrition labels to identify these products.

➢ Added sugars can be hidden in unexpected foods, such as sauces and items marketed as "healthy," like granola bars.

➢ While these foods are typically enjoyed during holidays and celebrations, it's crucial to consume them in moderation.

AVOID THESE FOODS:

- Cakes
- Candy
- Cereals
- Cookies
- Flavored low-fat or fat-free yogurts
- Granola and Granola bars
- Instant oatmeals
- Jellies
- Juices
- Lemonade
- Pies and cobblers
- Sauces: BBQ, ketchup, fat-free salad dressings, sriracha, teriyaki
- Energy drinks, Soft drinks and Sports drinks

REMEMBER!

Simple carbohydrates and overconsumption of refined grain products are the main factors contributing to NAFLD.

PROTEIN IS ESSENTIAL FOR THE BODY

Protein is vital for maintaining the health of our muscles, bones, blood, and skin.

Opt for plant-based protein, lean animal protein, or select dairy items.

Avoid deli meats, cured meats, and fried meat, as they tend to be higher in sodium and may contribute to high blood pressure.

Aim to include baked or broiled fish in your diet at least twice a week. Fish is a lean protein that can help decrease inflammation in the liver.

Reduce your consumption of red meat. When consuming red meat, opt for whole cuts and avoid processed varieties. You can still enjoy red meat occasionally, but limit it to one or two days per week.

- SELECT THESE PROTEIN TYPES:

- ANIMAL SOURCES: Lean beef (90%) Cod, Salmon, Skinless poultry, Eggs Tilapia, Tuna (steak or water-packed))

- PLANT PROTEINS:, Edamame, Tofu, Lentils, Nuts & seeds, Beans Nut butters, Tempeh,

LIMIT THESE TYPES OF PROTEINS:

Chorizo, Corned beef, Bacon Fried meats (fried chicken, chicken nuggets chicken fried steak), Hot dogs, Deli meats,Jerky, Pepperoni, Sausage

DAIRY, AN ALTERNATIVE SOURCE OF PROTEIN

Dairy products serve as another beneficial source of protein and can be incorporated into your diet in moderation.

Dairy also provides essential calcium, crucial for maintaining bone health.

It's advisable to steer clear of flavored, non-fat, or low-fat yogurts, as they frequently contain additional sugars that can contribute to health issues. Instead, opt for plain yogurt varieties or those labeled as unsweetened to minimize sugar intake and make a healthier choice for your diet.

Enjoy cheese in moderation, opting for unprocessed varieties, and being mindful not to overindulge.

SELECT THESE DAIRY ITEMS:

- Cottage cheese
- Skim or 2% Milk
- Greek yogurt

CHEESES: Ricotta (better tolerated because it's made from whey) Parmesan preferably aged over 24 months) Blue cheese, Cheddar, Mozzarella, Swiss, Feta, Goat cheese.

LIMIT THESE DAIRY ITEMS:

- Butter/margarine and Buttermilk
- Custard
- Flavored low-fat or non-fat yogurts
- Flavored creamers
- Heavy cream and Ice cream

- Sour cream

- CHEESES: Queso fresco American, Velveeta, Cream cheese

ARE FATS IMPORTANT FOR OUR HEALTH?

Dietary fats play a critical role in overall health, serving as a vital source of energy and aiding in the absorption of essential nutrients. However, it's essential to make informed choices when incorporating fats into your diet.

Instead of shying away from fats altogether, prioritize sources rich in omega-3 fatty acids, renowned for their numerous health benefits, including cardiovascular support and inflammation reduction. Keep in mind that while omega-3 fatty acids may not always be explicitly listed on nutrition labels, they are commonly found in fatty fish like salmon, walnuts, and flaxseeds.

Be cautious of products labeled as "fat-free" or "low-fat," as they often compensate for reduced fat content by adding sugars or other unhealthy ingredients. Additionally, steer clear of trans fats, which are commonly disguised on ingredient lists as "partially hydrogenated oils" or "hydrogenated oils." These fats, prevalent in commercially baked goods and fried foods, pose significant health risks and should be avoided whenever possible.

CHOOSE THESE TYPES OF FAT-CONTAINING FOODS:

- Avocados

- Canola oil

- Edamame

- Eggs

- Extra virgin olive oil

- Fatty fish (salmon, tuna)

- Full-fat yogurt

- Olives

- Whole nuts & seeds

- Nut & seed butters

LIMIT THESE TYPES OF FAT-CONTAINING FOODS:

- Margarine

- Fast-foods

- Fried foods

- Fish oil supplements (unless prescribed by your doctor)

- Ice cream

- Palm oil

- Processed snack foods

- Mayonnaise

- Some peanut butters (check the fat content)

- Store-bought salad dressings

SELECTING BEVERAGES

Hydration is paramount for maintaining good health, given that your body primarily consists of water.

Steer clear of sugar-sweetened beverages, as the sugars they contain are metabolized into fat upon reaching the liver, potentially exacerbating NAFLD.

Steering clear of alcohol is paramount, as it can exacerbate liver damage. Switching from sugary drinks might require a gradual adjustment period for your palate to adapt.

Patience is key as you acclimate to less sugar, eventually finding overly sweetened beverages unappealing.

CHOOSE THESE BEVERAGES:

- Black coffee

- Unsweetened hot or iced tea

- Water

- Craving Carbonation?

- If you're in need of fizz, consider seltzer water.

Yearning for Flavor?

Enhance your beverage with fresh or frozen fruit.

Sweetening Your Coffee?

Experiment with adding cinnamon, cocoa powder, or nutmeg for a flavorful twist.

PART

3

METHODS TO CRAFT FLAVORFUL VEGETABLE DISHES

ROASTING

- Utilizes high heat to achieve crispness in vegetables.

- Suitable for nearly any type of vegetable.

- Consider employing this method when preparing asparagus, Brussels sprouts, broccoli, carrots, sweet potatoes, bell peppers, onions, or zucchini.

Cooking Instructions:

1. Preheat the oven to 415°F.

2. In a spacious mixing bowl, blend oil, spices, and vegetables, ensuring an even coating.

3. Line a large sheet pan with parchment paper and arrange the vegetables, ensuring they are not overcrowded.

4. Roast for 15–20 minutes, pausing midway to stir the vegetables.

HELPFUL TIPS:

General guideline: Use 1 tablespoon of oil for every pound of raw vegetables (approximately 4–6 cups).

Avoid excessive oil: Using too much oil can result in soggy and less appetizing vegetables.

Uniformity in cutting: Cut vegetables into uniform sizes to ensure even cooking.

Prevent overcrowding: Arrange vegetables on the pan without overcrowding to ensure proper roasting.

SAUTÉING

- Utilizes high heat and a minimal amount of oil to swiftly cook vegetables while preserving their texture and flavor.

- Most effective for less dense vegetables such as onions, spinach, kale, mushrooms, and bell peppers.

Preparation:

1. Warm a spacious pan on medium to high heat.

2. Add a small amount of oil, just enough to lightly coat the bottom of the pan (approximately 2 teaspoons).

3. Once the oil is hot, add the vegetables, ensuring not to overcrowd the pan; you should hear a sizzle upon adding them.

4. Keep the vegetables in motion and cook until they are lightly browned and thoroughly cooked.

HELPFUL TIPS:

Remember that "sauté" translates to "to jump," so ensure that vegetables are continuously moving while cooking.

Dice vegetables or slice them thinly to promote even cooking.

Exercise caution with oil usage; excessive oil may result in pan-frying rather than sautéing the vegetables.

BLANCHING

Blanching is a culinary technique that entails submerging vegetables in boiling water for a short period, followed by rapid cooling to preserve their vibrant color and crisp texture. This method works exceptionally well with vegetables like broccoli, sugar snap peas, cauliflower, edamame, and green beans, ensuring they retain their optimal taste and appearance

Cooking Instructions:

1. Bring salted water to a rolling boil in a large pot.

2. Cut vegetables into evenly sized pieces and add them to the boiling water, cooking for approximately 2–4 minutes.

3. Remove vegetables promptly and transfer them into an ice bath or rinse them under cold water for a similar duration as the cooking time.

4. Pat dry the blanched vegetables using a dish or paper towel.

HELPFUL TIPS:

Ideal for those who prefer cooked vegetables over raw.

Can be used to prepare salads or snacks.

Cooking time may vary based on the type and size of the vegetable, so avoid overcooking.

This technique is useful for preserving excess vegetables by freezing them for later use.

GRILLING

- Utilizes direct heat to impart a smoky flavor to vegetables.

- Experiment with this method on eggplant, zucchini, mushrooms, onions, peppers, tomatoes, broccoli, or cauliflower.

Cooking Instructions:

1. Preheat the grill to medium-high heat.

2. Slice vegetables to a uniform thickness, approximately ¼-inch thick, ensuring they are long enough not to fall through the grill grates.

3. Lightly coat vegetables with oil and season them according to your preference.

4. Place vegetables on the grill and close the lid.

5. Allow vegetables to cook undisturbed for 3–5 minutes on each side.

USEFUL SUGGESTIONS

Cooking duration may differ based on the type and thickness of the vegetable.

Consider creating vegetable skewers for a convenient grilling option.

Aim for vegetables to achieve a pleasant char without becoming excessively charred.

SIMPLE SUBSTITUTIONS FOR LIVER-FRIENDLY MEALS

✓ Swap Vegetable Cooking Oil for Canola Oil

✓ Replace Foods Fried with Flour with Corn Starch for Light Coating

✓ Substitute All-Purpose White Flour with 100% Whole Wheat Flour

✓ Opt for Plain Greek Yogurt Instead of Sour Cream

✓ Use Fresh Fruit Instead of Flavored Jelly or Syrup

✓ Utilize Herbs and Spices to Flavor Food

SIMPLE SUBSTITUTIONS FOR LIVER-FRIENDLY MEALS

Vegetable Cooking Oil	Canola Oil / Extra Virgin Olive Oil
Foods Fried with Flour	Use Corn Starch for Light Coating
All-Purpose White Flour	100% Whole Wheat Flour
Sour Cream	Plain Greek Yogurt
Flavored Jelly or Syrup	Fresh Fruit

SALT GUIDELINES

Be cautious of seasoning blends high in sodium content.

Employ herbs and spices separately or in a blend without extra salt.

Adjust salt levels to personal taste at the conclusion of cooking.

Enhance the flavor of your dishes with a variety of herbs and spices, including turmeric cumin, parsley, thyme, bay leaves, curry, red pepper sage, black pepper, garlic, cajun, ginger, turmeric, cayenne, basil, nutmeg, , cinnamon, cilantro, oregano, rosemary, and paprika.

GROCERY STORE GUIDELINES

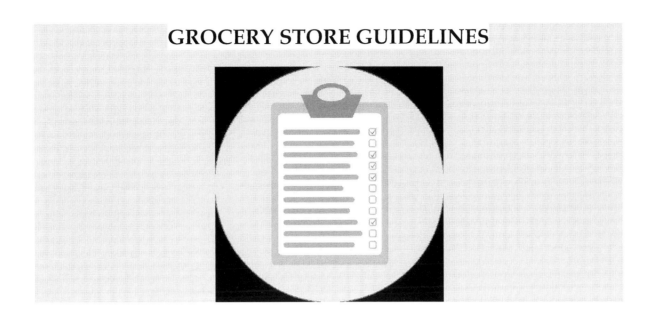

Opt for seasonal produce, often marked down for freshness.

Maintain a shopping list and adhere to it.

Strategize meal planning around weekly sale items, focusing on versatile ingredients.

Scrutinize nutrition labels for hidden sugars and trans fats, adhering to recommended serving sizes.

Prioritize vegetables, fruits, whole grains, and lean proteins like beans, fish, poultry, and nuts while steering clear of highly processed snacks.

Select canned goods labeled "low-sodium," "no salt added," or "packed in water"; if unavailable, rinse before use.

Consider frozen fruits and vegetables for cost-effectiveness and longevity, ensuring they're free of added sugars or juice, and rinsing canned fruit items.

Utilize canola oil for cooking as a budget-friendly alternative to olive oil, rich in omega-3 fatty acids beneficial for liver and heart health.

Minimize food waste through proper storage in the fridge and freezer.

PART
4

SAMPLE MEAL PLAN IDEAS

HOW SHOULD I STRUCTURE MY PLATE?

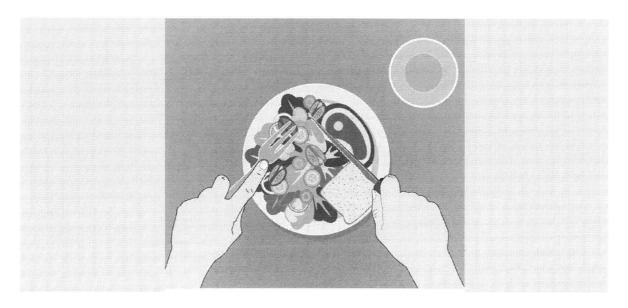

A key takeaway is to incorporate vegetables into every meal.

Ideally, each meal should encompass various food groups. Employing the plate method facilitates visualizing these groups and ensuring appropriate portion sizes. While the combination of foods—such as incorporating vegetables into sandwiches, soups, or pasta—may not perfectly reflect the depicted plate, it still contributes to a balanced diet.

BREAKFAST

Two Egg Breakfast Scramble

Size: One

INGREDIENTS

2 Eggs

½ Tbsp Canola oil, divided

1 cup non-starchy vegetables: bell pepper, mushroom, onion, spinach, tomato, or any listed on part 2

. *Choose as many of these vegetables as you like to form the base of your dish. Feel free to mix and match to create a combination that suits your taste preferences*

COOKING INSTRUCTIONS

1. Heat ¼ tbsp canola oil in a non-stick pan over medium heat.

2. Introduce the chosen vegetables to the skillet and sauté for approximately 5 minutes. Should you opt for spinach, incorporate it during the final minute of cooking..

3. Enhance the flavor of your vegetables by seasoning them with a variety of herbs and spices according to your taste preferences. Experiment with a diverse range of seasonings such as basil, oregano, thyme, rosemary, garlic, paprika, or cumin to add depth and complexity to your dish..

4. In a separate pan, cook the eggs in your preferred style, using the remaining canola oil.

5. Top the vegetable skillet with the cooked eggs and any suggested toppings.

Top It! Select a Grain or Fruit Option

Opt for one or combine multiple options:
¼ cup Cheddar or low-part-skim mozzarella cheese
½ cup cooked beans
¼ whole avocado, sliced
2, 6-inch corn tortillas
1 slice of 100% whole-wheat bread
Fresh salsa
¾ cup berries (choose from blackberries, blueberries, strawberries, or raspberries)

DAY 1: SIMPLE AND QUICK MENU

LUNCH

Crispy Chicken Salad

Servings Size: One

INGREDIENTS

1 chicken breast (4-6 oz)

1 Tbsp corn starch

½ Tbsp canola oil

2-3 cups dark leafy greens (such as bok choy, collard greens, kale, romaine, spinach, or swiss chard)

1 cup of any non-starchy vegetables, sliced

COOKING INSTRUCTIONS

1. Slice the chicken breast into ½-inch thick pieces.
2. In a small mixing bowl, combine corn starch and your choice of seasonings to flavor the chicken.
3. Add the chicken slices to the bowl, cover, and toss until the chicken is lightly coated.
4. Heat canola oil in a non-stick pan over medium heat and add the seasoned chicken.
5. Cook the chicken until it achieves a golden brown hue and is completely cooked, reaching an internal temperature of 165°F.
6. Prepare your salad base using a pre-made mix or create your own. Use any dark leafy greens and top with your choice of non-starchy vegetables.

Top It! Choose One Grain or Fruit

Select one or combine several:
Choose 1-2 Fat-Based Items:
5 olives
¼ cup nuts or seeds
¼ avocado, sliced
¼ cup cheese of your choice (see options on p. 17)
Dress Your Salad:
Toss salad with 2 Tbsp of dressing:

DAY 1: SIMPLE AND QUICK MENU

DINNER

Baked Fish and Roasted Vegetables

Servings Size: One

INGREDIENTS

Fish (4-6 oz) Catfish or Salmon, Cod, Tilapia

1 Tbsp canola oil

1/2 pint tomatoes

5-6 stalks asparagus, cut into 1-inch pieces

Seasoning Blends:

Orange Paprika:

1 Tbsp orange juice, ½ tsp paprika, ½ tsp dried dill,

Italian Blend:

1 Tbsp lime juice, 1 tsp dried rosemary, 1 tsp dried oregano, 1 tsp dried basil

Cilantro grapefruit

1 Tbsp grapefruit juice, 2 garlic cloves, minced, ¼ white onion, diced, 1 Tbsp fresh cilantro or ½ Tbsp dried cilantro,

¼ tsp chili powder and salt to taste

1. ## COOKING NSTRUCTIONS

2. Preheat your oven to 390°F.
3. Place the fish fillet on a large piece of aluminum foil.
4. In a large mixing bowl, mix canola oil with one of the seasoning blends.
5. Use half of the oil and seasoning mixture to coat the top of the fish.
6. Add the tomatoes and asparagus to the mixing bowl and coat them with the remaining oil blend.
7. Place the seasoned vegetables on the aluminum foil alongside the fish, then fold the foil over to create a sealed packet.
8. Cook for about 20 minutes or until the vegetables are tender and the fish reaches an internal temperature of 140°F.

Choose One Grain or Dessert

Select one or combine several:
½ cup cooked beans
½ cup cooked brown or wild rice, seasoned to taste
¾ cup fresh fruit topped with 2 Tbsp whipped cream

DAY 2: SIMPLE AND QUICK MENU

BREAKFAST

Oatmeal

Size: One

INGREDIENTS

½ cup Dried oats

1 cup Water or milk

COOKING INSTRUCTIONS

For best results, opt for whole oats instead of instant microwaveable oatmeal packets. Heat the oats following the package directions, either using the microwave or cooking them on the stovetop.

Note that if you choose to cook the oatmeal in milk, it will serve as your protein portion.

Top It! Choose One Grain or Vegeteble

Customize your oatmeal with one grain and one vegetable option::
Opt for a quarter cup of nuts, preferably walnuts, almonds, or pecans.
Alternatively, select a quarter cup of mixed berries or half of a whole banana.
Add extra flavor with cinnamon, nutmeg, apple pie spice, or cocoa.
Additionally, cook an egg in any preferred style, or Incorporate half a cup of plain Greek yogurt., or Include half a cup of cottage cheese.
Serve with three to four ounces of lean breakfast meat, such as Canadian bacon, chicken sausage, or turkey bacon.
Enjoy half a small zucchini, sliced and sautéed or roasted, or Add four to six Brussels sprouts, quartered and sautéed or roasted.

To save time in the morning, prepare extra vegetables during the week to have them ready to add to your breakfast.

DAY 2: SIMPLE AND QUICK MENU

LUNCH

Crispy Sandwich

Servings Size: One

INGREDIENTS

2 slices of 100% whole-wheat bread

3-4 oz of meat, baked or grilled, options include chicken, fish, turkey, canned tuna, or lean beef

Assorted vegetable toppings, either cooked or raw, such as banana pepper, mushrooms, bell pepper, onion, cucumber, pickles, jalapeño, tomato, and lettuce

COOKING INSTRUCTIONS

1. Select 2 slices of 100% whole-wheat bread for the base of the sandwich.
2. Choose a 3-4 oz portion of meat, either baked or grilled, from options like chicken, fish, turkey, canned tuna, or lean beef.
3. Add assorted vegetable toppings, either cooked or raw, according to preference, such as banana pepper, mushrooms, bell pepper, onion, cucumber, pickles, jalapeño, tomato, and lettuce..

Enhance your vegetables by pairing them with a flavorful dip

Choose 1-2 fat-based items such as 1 oz of cheese (refer to page xx), ¼ of a whole avocado, 1 tablespoon of mayonnaise made with olive oil, or 2 tablespoons of hummus.
Select condiments to add flavor, choosing from options like hot sauce, mustard, spices/herbs, and vinegar.
Prepare a cup of sliced raw vegetables, such as bell pepper, carrot, celery, cucumber, and zucchini. Mix and match according to your preference.
Pair your vegetable selection with 2 tablespoons of your chosen dip, which could be hummus in any flavor, Greek yogurt ranch dip, homemade salad dressing, bean dip, or fresh salsa.

DINNER

Steak Tacos

Servings Size: One

INGREDIENTS

3-4 oz of your preferred protein, approximately the size of your palm and 1 inch thick. Options include:

- o Sirloin / Shrimp
- o Flank or skirt steak
- o Lean ground beef (85-90%)

½ tablespoon of canola oil

Spice Blend:

¼ teaspoon of chili powder

¼ teaspoon of onion powder

2 cloves of garlic, minced

2 tablespoons of pineapple juice (optional)

1 tablespoon of soy sauce

Juice of 1 lime

½ tablespoon of canola oil

COOKING INSTRUCTIONS

1. In a shallow dish, combine the spice blend ingredients. Mix in your preferred protein and let it marinate for 30 minutes at room temperature.
2. Warm up a cast iron skillet over medium-high heat and pour in some canola oil.
3. Place the marinated protein into the skillet. Adjust the cooking time based on the type of protein selected:
4. For steak cooked to medium, cook each side for approximately 5 minutes, flipping only once.
5. For lean beef, cook until it is fully browned or reaches an internal temperature of 160°F.
6. Shrimp usually take around 5 minutes to cook completely and should reach an internal temperature of 145°F...

Serve with:

Select one or combine several:
Diced tomato
Diced onion

Fresh salsa
Fajita vegetables
Shredded lettuce
Cilantro
Substitute for sour cream: 1 tablespoon of plain Greek yogurt
Queso fresco: ¼ cup

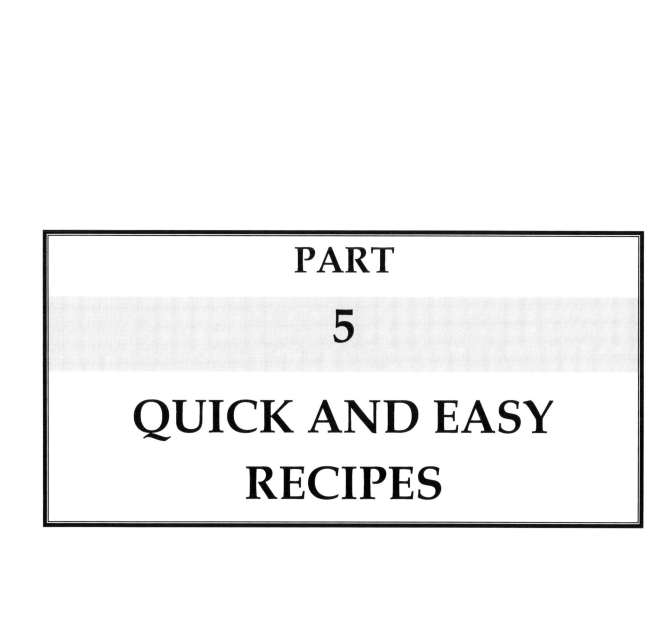

PART

5

QUICK AND EASY RECIPES

Breakfast

Cottage Cheese Pancakes

Prep Time
10 min

Cook Time
10 min

Servings
2

Ingredients
1/2 cup low-fat cottage cheese (or fat-free)
1/2 cup whole wheat flour (for extra fiber)
1/4 cup unsweetened almond milk (or other plant-based milk)
1 large egg white (to reduce fat content)
1 tbsp natural sweetener (e.g., stevia or monk fruit, optional)
1/2 tsp baking powder
1/2 tsp vanilla extract - a pinch of salt
1/2 cup fresh strawberries (sliced)

Preparation
Mix the wet ingredients: In a medium bowl, whisk together the low-fat cottage cheese, egg white, almond milk, and vanilla extract until smooth.

Mix dry ingredients: In a separate bowl, whisk together whole wheat flour, baking powder, sweetener (if using), and salt.

Prepare the batter: Gradually add the dry ingredients to the wet mixture, stirring just until combined. Adjust thickness with almond milk if needed.

Cook pancakes: Heat a non-stick skillet over medium heat, coat with cooking spray, and pour about 2 tablespoons of batter per pancake. Cook until bubbles form and edges are set (2-3 minutes), flip, and cook until golden, about 2 minutes more.

Serve: Stack the pancakes on a plate, top with fresh strawberry slices.

Nutrition: **|Calories: 190 | Fat: 3 g |Carbs: 19 g |Sugar:3 g |Protein: 14**

Green Omelette

Prep Time
10 min

Cook Time
10 min

Servings
1

Ingredients
2 eggs
1/6 cup milk
1/4 cup shredded cheese and 1/4 cup diced ham
1/4 cup diced bell pepper
1 tbsp extra virgin olive oil
A pinch of parsley chopped and salt to taste

Preparation
In a bowl, whisk together 2 eggs, 1/6 cup of milk, parsley, and salt to taste until well combined.

Heat a pan over medium heat and add a bit of oil to prevent sticking.

Pour the egg mixture into the pan and let it cook for a minute until it starts to set around the edges. Sprinkle shredded cheese, diced ham, and diced bell pepper evenly over one half of the omelette.

Fold the omelette in half over the filling and cook for another minute until the cheese has melted and the omelette is thoroughly cooked.

Then, carefully transfer the omelette to a plate and serve promptly.

Nutrition: |Calories: 224 | Fat: 15 g |Carbs: 4 g |Sugar:2 g |Protein: 18

Avocado and Egg Bowl

Prep Time	Cook Time	Servings
10 min	10 min	1

Ingredients
1/2 ripe avocados

2 large eggs

salt to taste

1 tbsp extra virgin olive oil

Fresh herbs (such as cilantro or parsley)

Preparation
Cut the ripe avocado in half and remove the pit. Scoop out some of the flesh from each avocado half to create a larger space for the eggs. Carefully crack an egg into each avocado half, keeping the yolk intact. Season the eggs with salt to taste.

Heat the olive oil in a skillet over medium heat

Cook for about 5-7 minutes, or until the egg whites are set but the yolks are still runny.

Carefully remove the avocado and egg halves from the skillet and place them on serving plates.

Garnish with freshly chopped herbs.

Nutrition: |Calories: 324 | Fat: 19 g |Carbs: 9 g |Sugar:2 g |Protein: 15

Egg-cellent Chicken Bites

Prep Time	Cook Time	Servings
10 min	10 min	1

Ingredients
3 ounces of chicken, cut into 1-inch pieces

2 eggs

salt to taste

1/4 cup shredded cheese

1 tbsp canola oil

turmeric to taste

Preparation
In a bowl, crack the eggs and beat them until well combined.

Season to taste with salt. Combine the shredded cheese with the beaten eggs, ensuring an even distribution.

In a skillet over medium heat, heat the canola oil. Cook the chicken pieces until browned and fully cooked, approximately 4-5 minutes.

Once cooked, pour the egg and cheese mixture over the chicken in the skillet. Sprinkle turmeric over the mixture for added flavor and color. Cook the mixture, stirring occasionally, until the eggs are fully set and the cheese is melted, approximately 3-4 minutes.

Remove the skillet from the stove and allow the mixture to cool slightly, giving it a moment to settle.

Serve hot.

Nutrition: |Calories: 236 | Fat: 14 g | Carbs: 2 g |Sugar:1 g |Protein: 16

Italian Style Eggs

Prep Time

5 min

Cook Time

8 min

Servings

1

Ingredients

2 large eggs

1/2 diced avocado

1 diced tomatoe

chopped basil

1 tbsp extra virgin olive oil

salt to taste

Preparation

Heat the extra-virgin olive oil in a nonstick pan.

Crack the eggs into the pan, add salt, and let them set.

Once set, scramble the eggs.

Plate the scrambled eggs and then add raw tomato pieces and fresh basil leaves for extra flavor and freshness.

Nutrition: |Calories: 305 | Fat: 14 g |Carbs: 6 g |Sugar:1 g |Protein: 16

Blueberry Flan

Prep Time
3 min

Cook Time
7 min

Servings
2

Ingredients
4 large eggs
1/2 cup of almond milk
1/2 cup of fresh blueberries
2 tbsp of erythritol or another low-carb sweetener ₁
1 tsp of vanilla extract
salt to tast
ground cinnamon to taste

Preparation

Preheat your oven to 350°F (175°C).

In a mixing bowl, whisk together the eggs, almond milk, erythritol, vanilla extract, and a pinch of salt until well combined.

Grease a small baking dish or ramekin with a little oil or butter.

Evenly distribute the fresh blueberries across the bottom of the baking dish. Pour the egg mixture over the blueberries. Lightly sprinkle ground cinnamon over the top.

Place the baking dish in the preheated oven and bake for approximately 7 minutes, or until the flan is firm and no longer jiggles in the center.

After baking, take the dish out of the oven and let it cool for a short while before serving.

This brief resting period allows the flavors to meld and ensures a more enjoyable dining experience.

Nutrition: | Calories: 160 | Fat: 8 g | Carbs: 6 g | Sugar:4 g | Protein: 9

Mini Cinnamon Biscuits

Prep Time
10 min

Cook Time
6 min

Servings
2

Ingredients
1/2 cup almond flour and 1/2 cup coconut flour
2 tbsp low-carb sweetener (such as erythritol)
1 tsp baking powder
1 egg
salt to taste
, 1/4 cup of canola oil
1 tsp vanilla extract
2 tsp ground cinnamon

Preparation
Start by preheating the oven to 350°F (175°C) and lining a baking sheet with parchment paper. In a mixing bowl, blend together the almond flour, coconut flour, low-carb sweetener, baking powder, and a pinch of salt. In a separate bowl, whisk together the egg, 1/4 cup of canola oil, and vanilla extract until thoroughly combined.

Mix the wet ingredients thoroughly into the dry ingredients until they are fully incorporated and a cohesive dough forms. Ensure that all the ingredients are well blended, as this will help create a consistent texture and flavor throughout the dough. Carefully fold in the ground cinnamon, ensuring it is evenly distributed throughout the dough.

Using your hands or a small scoop, form the dough into small, bite-sized biscuits and place them

Nutrition: |Calories: 230 | Fat: 16 g |Carbs: 6 g |Sugar:1 g |Protein: 9

Zucchini Pie

Prep Time
10 min

Cook Time
25 min

Servings
2

Ingredients

1/2 cups of almond flour
1/2 cup of shredded cheddar cheese
2 tablespoons of extra virgin olive oil
2 medium zucchinis, grated
4 large eggs
basil and dried garlic to taste
salt to taste

Preparation

Preheat your oven to 375°F (190°C) and grease a 9-inch pie dish.

In a bowl, mix together the almond flour, shredded cheddar cheese, and a pinch of salt. Incorporate the extra virgin olive oil until the mixture resembles coarse crumbs. Evenly distribute and press the almond flour mixture into the greased pie dish to form a solid crust foundation. In a separate large bowl, vigorously whisk the eggs until thoroughly beaten, ensuring a smooth consistency for the filling..

Add the grated zucchinis, dried basil, garlic powder, and a pinch of salt to the egg mixture. Stir until all ingredients are well incorporated.

Pour the zucchini and egg mixture over the crust in the pie dish, spreading it out evenly.

Bake in the preheated oven for 25 minutes, or until the top is golden brown and the center is set.

Let the zucchini pie cool for a few minutes before slicing and serving.

Nutrition: |Calories: 360 | Fat: 12 g |Carbs: 16 g |Sugar:3 g |Protein: 15

Breakfast Pizza

Prep Time
10 min

Cook Time
10 min

Servings
1

Ingredients
2 whole pitas
4 tablespoons sugar-free tomato sauce
1/2 cup shredded mozzarella cheese
1/2 cup chopped bell pepper, onion, and spinac
2 large eggs
1 tablespoon extra virgin olive oil
salt to taste

Preparation

Preheat your oven to 375°F (190°C).

Place the pitas on a baking sheet and spread 1 tablespoon of sugar-free tomato sauce on each pita.

Sprinkle shredded mozzarella cheese on each pita.

Evenly distribute the chopped bell pepper, onion, and spinach over the cheese.

Drizzle 1 tablespoon of extra virgin olive oil over the toppings.

Add salt to taste.

Place the baking sheet in the oven and bake for 10 minutes, or until the cheese is melted and bubbly.

Take out from the oven, allow it to cool for a brief moment, and then serve while still hot.

Nutrition: |Calories: 354 | Fat: 23 g |Carbs: 8 g |Sugar:2 g |Protein: 24

VEGETABLES

Roasted Broccoli with Garlic and Lemon

Prep Time
5 min

Cook Time
20 min

Servings
2

Ingredients
1 head of broccoli, cut into florets
2 tablespoons extra virgin olive oil
3 cloves garlic, minced
Zest of 1 lemon
1 tablespoon lemon juice
Salt, to taste
Grated Parmesan cheese (optional, for serving)

Preparation
Preheat the oven to 425°F (220°C).

Prepare the broccoli by rinsing the florets under cold water and drying them with a kitchen towel.

Trim any tough stems and cut the broccoli into bite-sized pieces. In a large mixing bowl, coat the broccoli florets with olive oil, minced garlic, lemon zest, lemon juice, salt, and pepper.

Ensure the florets are evenly coated. Arrange the seasoned broccoli in a single layer on a baking sheet lined with parchment paper or aluminum foil. Roast in the preheated oven for 15-20 minutes until tender and slightly charred.

Once roasted, transfer the broccoli to a serving dish.

Nutrition: |Calories: 126 | Fat: 5 g |Carbs: 15 g |Sugar:2 g |Protein: 10 g

Baked Sweet Potato

Prep Time
10 min

Cook Time
30 min

Servings
2

Ingredients
2 medium sweet potatoes
2 tablespoons extra virgin olive oil
1 teaspoon garlic powder
1 teaspoon paprika
Salt and pepper, to taste
Fresh parsley, chopped (for garnish)

Preparation
Preheat the oven to 400°F (200°C).

Scrub the sweet potatoes clean under running water and pat them dry.

Puncture the sweet potatoes with a toothpick or fork to allow steam to escape. Then, mix extra virgin olive oil, , paprika, salt, pepper and garlic powder together before rubbing the mixture over the sweet potatoes

 Arrange them on a baking sheet and bake for 40-45 minutes until tender.

Let them cool, then slice and fluff the flesh with a fork.

Sprinkle with fresh parsley before serving.

Nutrition: |Calories: 210 | Fat: 10 g |Carbs: 38 g |Sugar:9 g |Protein: 8 g

Baked Brussels Sprouts

Prep Time
10 min

Cook Time
20 min

Servings
2

Ingredients

1 pound Brussels sprouts, trimmed and halved

2 tablespoons olive oil

2 cloves garlic, minced

1 teaspoon Dijon mustard

1 tablespoon balsamic vinegar

Salt and pepper, to taste

Preparation

Preheat the oven to 400°F (200°C).

Prepare the Brussels sprouts by rinsing them under cold water and drying them with a kitchen towel.

Trim the ends and cut them in half lengthwise. In a large mixing bowl, combine the halved Brussels sprouts with olive oil, minced garlic, Dijon mustard, balsamic vinegar, salt, and pepper.

Ensure the Brussels sprouts are thoroughly coated with the mixture by tossing them until every surface is evenly covered.

Transfer the seasoned Brussels sprouts to a baking dish or a baking sheet lined with parchment paper, arranging them in a single layer with the cut side down for even cooking.

Place the baking dish in the preheated oven and bake for 20-25 minutes, or until the Brussels sprouts are tender and caramelized.

Once baked, remove the Brussels sprouts from the oven and transfer them to a serving dish.

Nutrition: | Calories: 174 | Fat: 5 g | Carbs: 10 g | Sugar: 4 g | Protein: 4 g

Stir-Fried Vegetables with Ginger and Garlic

Prep Time
10 min

Cook Time
10 min

Servings
2

Ingredients
1 cup broccoli florets
1 small carrot, julienned or thinly sliced
1/2 red bell pepper, sliced
1 small zucchini, sliced
1/2 cup snow peas (or green beans)
2 cloves garlic, minced
1-inch piece of fresh ginger, minced
1 tbsp soy sauce
1 tsp sesame oil (optional, for flavor)
1 tbsp avocado oil for cooking
Green onions or fresh cilantro for garnish (optional)
1 tsp sesame seeds (optional for garnish)

Preparation
Prepare the ingredients: Wash and chop all the vegetables, making sure to cut them into even pieces for quick and uniform cooking. Mince the garlic and ginger.

Heat the oil: Warm avocado oil in a large non-stick skillet or wok over medium-high heat.

Stir-fry aromatics: Add garlic and ginger to the hot oil, stir-fry for 1 minute until fragrant, being careful not to burn them.

Cook the vegetables: Add broccoli, carrots, bell pepper, zucchini, and snow peas to the skillet.

Stir-fry for about 5-6 minutes, stirring frequently, until the vegetables are crisp-tender. Add soy sauce: Stir in the low-sodium soy sauce (and sesame oil if using) and cook for another minute, tossing the vegetables to coat them evenly in the sauce.

Serve: Remove the vegetables from the heat and garnish with sesame seeds, fresh cilantro, or green onions if desired. Serve as a main dish with a side of quinoa or brown rice, or as a side dish to lean protein.

Nutrition: |Calories: 140 | Fat: 4 g |Carbs: 14 g |Sugar: 4 g |Protein: 8 g

CEREAL BASED DISHES

Rosemary and Parmesan Lentil Croquettes

Prep Time
5 min

Cooking time
20 min

Servings
2 Pieces

Ingredients
1 cup cooked lentils
1/4 cup breadcrumbs
1/4 cup grated Parmesan cheese
1 tablespoon chopped fresh rosemary
1 clove garlic, minced
1 egg, beaten
Salt and pepper, to taste
2 tablespoons extra virgin olive oil (for cooking)

Preparation

Begin by boiling the lentils in water according to package instructions until tender. Once cooked, drain the excess water and set them aside to cool.

Mix Ingredients: In a large mixing bowl, combine the cooked lentils, breadcrumbs, grated Parmesan cheese, chopped fresh rosemary, minced garlic, beaten egg, salt, and pepper.

Using a fork or your hands, thoroughly mix all the ingredients until they are well combined.

Take small portions of the lentil mixture and shape them into small croquettes or patties; this recipe should yield about 4 croquettes.

In a generously sized non-stick skillet, warm the olive oil over medium heat until it reaches an optimal temperature for cooking

Once the oil is hot, carefully place the lentil croquettes in the pan, leaving some space between each one.

Cook for approximately 4-5 minutes on each side, or until they turn golden brown and crispy.

Once the croquettes are cooked through and crispy on the outside, transfer them to a serving plate.

You can serve them hot as they are or with your preferred dipping sauce on the side.

Nutrition: Calories: 235 | Fat: 11 g | Carbs: 16 g |Sugar: 2 g | Protein: 12

Lentil Tacos

Prep   Time
5 min

Cooking time
20 min

Servings
2 Pieces

Ingredients

1 cup cooked lentils

1 tbsp canola

oil

1/4 cup vegetable broth or water

1 onion, diced

2 cloves garlic, minced

1 tsp ground cumin

1 tsp chili powder

1/2 tsp paprika

Salt and pepper, to taste

4 tortillas

Toppings of your choice:

, salsa, tomatoes, lettuce, avocado slices, etc.

Preparation

begin boiling lentils in water according to package instructions until tender. Remove any excess water from the lentils and set them aside.

In a large skillet, warm the canola oil over medium heat.

Add the diced onion and minced garlic, then sauté until they become soft and aromatic, usually about 3-4 minutes.

Next, add the cooked lentils to the skillet along with the ground cumin, chili powder, paprika, salt, and pepper and stir well.

Pour vegetable broth or water into the skillet and stir to combine.

Let the mixture simmer for approximately 5-7 minutes, or until most of the liquid has evaporated and the lentils are heated through.

Meanwhile, warm the tortillas in a dry skillet or microwave until they become soft and pliable.

Assemble Tacos: Spoon the lentil mixture onto the warmed tortillas, dividing it evenly among them. Top each taco with your desired toppings, such as diced tomatoes, shredded lettuce, avocado slices, salsa, etc.

Serve.

Nutrition: Calories: 205 | Fat: 5 g | Carbs: 23 g |Sugar: 2 g | Protein: 12

Chickpea and Zucchini Chips

Prep   Time
5 min

Cooking time
20 min

Servings
2 Pieces

Ingredients
1 cup chickpeas (drained and rinsed)
2 medium zucchinis (sliced)
2 tbsp canola oil

1 tsp paprika
1 tsp garlic powder
1 tsp salt
1/2 tsp black pepper

Preparation

Preheat your oven to 400°F (200°C) and line a baking sheet with parchment paper or aluminum foil.

Prepare the Chickpeas: Dry off the chickpeas using a paper towel to eliminate any excess moisture. Place them in a bowl and add a tablespoon of olive oil. Sprinkle with garlic powder, paprika, salt, and pepper. Mix well to ensure even coating. Spread the seasoned chickpeas onto one side of the prepared baking sheet. Place the baking sheet in the preheated oven and roast for 20-25 minutes, or until crispy, flipping them halfway through.

While the chickpeas are roasting, thinly slice the zucchini using either a sharp knife or a mandoline slicer. Transfer the zucchini slices to a bowl and drizzle them with the remaining tablespoon of canola oil. Add salt and pepper, and toss to coat evenly.

Bake the Zucchini: Arrange the seasoned zucchini slices in a single layer on the other side of the baking sheet. Place the sheet back in the oven and bake for 10-15 minutes, or until the zucchini turns golden brown and crispy, flipping them halfway through.

Serve: Once both the chickpeas and zucchini chips achieve a crispy, golden texture, take them out of the oven.

Nutrition: Calories: 205 | Fat: 12 g | Carbs: 20 g | Sugar: 4 g | Protein: 10

MEAT BASED

DISHES

Savory Herb-Crusted Beef

Prep Time
5 min

Cook Time
12 min

Servings
2

Ingredients
2 beef medallions (each about 4 ounces)
2 tablespoons canola oil
1 tablespoon Dijon mustard
2 cloves garlic, minced
1 teaspoon dried rosemary
1 teaspoon dried thyme
Salt and pepper to taste

Preparation
In a small bowl, mix the minced garlic, dried rosemary, dried thyme, salt, and pepper. Evenly coat both sides of the beef medallions with Dijon mustard, then press the herb mixture onto the surface.

Heat the canola oil in a skillet over medium-high heat and carefully place the beef medallions in the pan, searing them for about 2 to 3 minutes on each side until a golden crust forms.

Lower the heat and continue cooking for another couple of minutes or until the desired degree of doneness is reached.

Serve the herb-crusted beef medallions with roasted vegetables or a fresh salad for a flavorful and balanced meal.

Nutrition | Calories: 196 | Fat: 9 g | Carbs: 1 g | Sugar: 0 g | Protein: 29 g

Grilled Meats with Tzatziki Sauce

Prep Time
10 min

Cook Time
15 min

Servings
2

Ingredients
For the Grilled Meats:
2 beef steaks
2 tablespoons canola oil
2 cloves garlic, minced
1 tablespoon lemon juice
1 teaspoon dried oregano and thyme
salt to taste

For the Tzatziki Sauce:
1 cup Greek yogurt
1/2 cucumber, grated and drained
2 cloves garlic, minced
1 tablespoon lemon juice
1 tablespoon canola oil
1 tablespoon fresh dill, chopped (or 1 teaspoon dried dill)
Salt and pepper to taste

Preparation

Arrange the meat pieces in a small bowl and coat them evenly with a mixture of canola oil, minced garlic, lemon juice, dried oregano, dried thyme, and salt.

Let the meat marinate for at least 30 minutes to allow the flavors to meld together.

Preheat the grill to medium-high heat and grill the meat for approximately 4 minutes on each side, or until it reaches your preferred level of doneness.

Tzatziki Sauce: In a medium-sized bowl, combine Greek yogurt, grated cucumber (ensure to squeeze out excess water), minced garlic, lemon juice, canola oil, chopped dill, salt, and pepper.

Ensure thorough mixing of all ingredients until a homogeneous mixture is achieved. After preparing the sauce, cover it securely and transfer it to the refrigerator, allowing it to chill for at least 30 minutes.

Serve the grilled meats straight from the grill, accompanied by a generous serving of tzatziki sauce.

Nutrition: |Calories: 196 | Fat: 5 g |Carbs: 24 g |Sugar:5 g | Protein: 16 g

Super Crispy Chicken Wings

Prep Time
5 min

Cooking time
25 min

Servings
2

Ingredients
4 chicken wings
Salt to taste
Garlic powder to taste
Paprika to taste
1 teaspoon onion powder
2 tablespoons extra virgin olive oil

For the Anchovy Salad:
4 anchovy fillets, chopped
1 cup mixed salad greens,
1 cucumber and 1/4 red onion, thinly sliced
2 tablespoons lemon juice
1 tablespoon extra virgin olive oil
salt to taste

Preparation
Preheat your oven to 425°F (220°C).

In a large mixing bowl, toss the chicken wings with salt, garlic powder, paprika, and onion powder.

Drizzle with extra virgin olive oil and mix until the wings are evenly coated. Arrange the seasoned wings on a parchment-lined baking sheet.

Bake in the preheated oven for 25 minutes, flipping halfway through, until they are crispy and golden brown.

Meanwhile, prepare the salad by combining mixed greens, sliced cucumber, cherry tomatoes, red onion, and chopped anchovy fillets in a large bowl. In a separate small bowl, whisk together lemon juice, extra virgin olive oil, salt, and pepper to make the dressing.

Dress the salad and serve it alongside the chicken wings.

Nutrition: | Calories: 357 | Fat: 19 g | Carbs: 3 g | Sugar: 1 g | Protein: 25 g

Super Chicken Tenders

Prep Time
10 min

Cooking time
20 min

Servings
2

Ingredients

2 boneless, skinless chicken breasts, cut into tenders

1 teaspoon turmeric powder

1/2 teaspoon garlic powder

1/2 teaspoon paprika

salt to taste

1/2 cup all-purpose flour

1 large egg, beaten

1 cup panko breadcrumbs

2 tablespoons canola oil

Preparation

Start by preheating the oven to 200°C and lining a baking sheet with baking paper. In a bowl, combine turmeric powder, garlic powder, paprika, and salt to create a harmonious mix of flavors. Sprinkle this seasoning mixture evenly over the chicken fillets, ensuring each piece is thoroughly coated for maximum flavor infusion.

Next, prepare three shallow dishes: one with whole wheat flour, another with beaten eggs, and the third with panko breadcrumbs. Dip each chicken piece first in the flour, then in the egg, and finally coat it with breadcrumbs, applying light pressure to ensure the crumbs adhere well.

Arrange the chicken pieces in a single layer on the prepared baking sheet, making sure they are evenly spaced to allow for even cooking. For a crispier texture, lightly drizzle the chicken pieces with extra-virgin olive oil before baking. Bake for about 8 minutes, then turn the chicken pieces with a spatula to ensure even cooking and crispiness. Continue cooking for another 8 minutes or until fully cooked and golden brown.

At this point, your Super Chicken Tenders are ready to be served immediately with your favorite sauce or a side salad.

Nutrition: | Calories: 335 | Fat: 20 g | Carbs: 9 g | Sugar: 1 g | Protein: 29 g

Steak Bites and Mushrooms

Prep Time
5 min

Cooking time
15 min

Servings
2

Ingredients

1/2 pound steak (such as sirloin or ribeye), cut into 1-inch cubes

2 cups mushrooms, sliced

2 tablespoons canola oil

1 teaspoon garlic powder

1/2 teaspoon onion powder

1/2 teaspoon paprika

1/2 teaspoon salt (or to taste)

2 tablespoons fresh parsley, chopped (optional, for garnish)

Preparation

Heat a large skillet over medium-high heat and add 1 tablespoon of canola oil. Add the meat morsels along with the garlic, onion, and paprika. Allow the morsels to sear for about 5 minutes, then add salt. Once cooked, transfer the morsels to a plate.

In the same pan, add the remaining extra-virgin olive oil and introduce the sliced mushrooms, letting them cook for about 10 minutes. Return the meat morsels to the skillet with the mushrooms, sautéing over medium-low heat for another two minutes.

If necessary, adjust the seasoning with more salt, and add finely chopped fresh parsley.

Enjoy the steak and mushroom bites!

Nutrition: |Calories: 235 | Fat: 15 g |Carbs: 4 g |Sugar:2 g |Protein: 21 g

English Roast Beef with Citronette

Prep Time
10 min

Cook Time
30 min

Servings
4

Ingredients
2.2 pounds beef sirloin
1 tablespoon coarse salt
1/4 cup fresh sage leaves
1/4 cup fresh rosemary leaves
2 tablespoons extra-virgin olive oil
1/2 teaspoon yellow mustard powder

For the Citronette
Juice of 1 lemon
3 tablespoons extra-virgin olive oil
1 teaspoon mustard

Preparation

Start by washing and patting dry the aromatic herbs with absorbent paper. Place the salt, rosemary, and sage into a food processor. Blend everything until fine, then add the mustard powder and blend again. For convenience, transfer the rub into another bowl. Take a pinch of the rub and use it to season the beef, massaging it well with your hands to ensure even coverage. Set aside the remaining rub for later use.

Heat a drizzle of olive oil in a pan and sear the beef well on all sides, being careful not to pierce the meat. Once the meat is well browned, transfer it back to the cutting board. You can mix a half tablespoon of water into the herb salt and mix it well. Use this mixture to cover the top of the roast, first placing it in the center with a spoon, then spreading and pressing it gently with your hands to make it adhere better.

Place the seasoned beef on a rack inside a roasting pan, ensuring it doesn't touch the bottom of the pan for even cooking. Cook in a preheated, fan-assisted oven at 420°F on the middle rack for 15 minutes. After this time, lower the temperature to 350°F and cook for another 10-12 minutes. The internal temperature of the meat should be between 118-126°F depending on whether you prefer it more rare or pink.

For the Citronette: mix the lemon juice, mustard, and extra-virgin olive oil in a bowl, whisking until you achieve a stable emulsion.

Once the cooking time is up, remove the meat from the oven and let it rest. Slice the meat and prepare to plate. On each plate, place a couple of slices of meat, drizzle a bit of Citronette over the top, and garnish with a sprig of rosemary.

Enjoy your English-style roast beef!

Nutrition: |Calories: 246 | Fat: 15 g |Carbs: 1 g |Sugar: 0 g |Protein: 26 g

Lamb Burgers

Prep Time
10 min

Cook Time
10 min

Servings
2

Ingredients
1/2 pound ground lamb
1/4 cup finely chopped onion
1 clove garlic, minced
1 tablespoon fresh parsley, chopped
1 teaspoon ground cumin
1/2 teaspoon ground turmeric
1/2 teaspoon salt
1 tablespoon extra virgin olive oil

Preparation

In a large bowl, combine the ground lamb, chopped onion, minced garlic, parsley, ground cumin, ground turmeric and salt.

Combine the ingredients thoroughly until uniformly mixed. Shape the mixture into two equal-sized patties, each about 3/4 inch thick. In a generously sized skillet, warm up the olive oil over medium heat until it shimmers. When the oil is hot enough, carefully place the lamb patties in the skillet. Allow them to cook undisturbed for about 6 to 7 minutes on each side, aiming for an internal temperature of approximately 160°F (71°C) to achieve a medium level of doneness.

Depending on your personal preference, you can tailor the cooking time accordingly for a desired level of doneness. Once the lamb burgers are cooked to perfection, carefully remove them from the skillet and set them aside for a brief rest.

Serve the lamb burgers on toasted buns with your desired toppings and condiments for an extra burst of flavor. Enjoy your delicious Lamb Burger!

Nutrition: |Calories: 446 | Fat: 23 g |Carbs: 10 g |Sugar: 2 g |Protein: 31 g

Mediterranean Veal Medallions

Prep Time

5 min

Cook Time

15 min

Servings

2

Ingredients

1/2 pound veal medallions

1 tablespoon extra virgin olive oil

1 clove garlic, minced

1/2 cup cherry tomatoes, halved

1/4 cup Kalamata olives, pitted and halved

1/4 cup crumbled feta cheese

1 teaspoon dried oregano

1/2 lemon, juiced

Salt and pepper to taste

Fresh basil leaves, for garnish

Preparation

Mince the garlic, halve the cherry tomatoes and olives, and crumble the feta cheese.

Season both sides of the veal medallions with salt, pepper, and dried oregano. Heat extra virgin olive oil in a large skillet over medium-high heat.

Add the veal medallions and cook for approximately 3-4 minutes on each side until they are browned to your liking.

Set them aside. In the same skillet, add minced garlic and sauté for about 30 seconds until it becomes fragrant.

Incorporate the cherry tomatoes and Kalamata olives, cooking for roughly 2-3 minutes until the tomatoes begin to soften.

Return the veal medallions to the skillet. Drizzle lemon juice over them and sprinkle crumbled feta cheese on top.

Cook for an additional 1-2 minutes until the cheese slightly melts.

Garnish with fresh basil leaves and serve promptly.Enjoy this quick and flavorful Mediterranean-inspired veal dish with a side of your favorite vegetables or a simple green salad.

Nutrition |Calories: 335 | Fat: 19 g |Carbs: 9 g |Sugar: 5 g |Protein: 23 g

Herb-Crusted Lamb Chops

Prep Time
5 min

Cook Time
20 min

Servings
2

Ingredients

4 lamb chops

2 tablespoons extra virgin olive oil

1 tablespoon Dijon mustard

1/4 cup breadcrumbs

1/4 cup grated Parmesan cheese

1 teaspoon dried thyme

1 teaspoon dried rosemary

1 clove garlic, minced

Salt to taste

Preparation

Season the lamb chops with salt and pepper on both sides.

In a small bowl, combine the breadcrumbs, grated Parmesan cheese, dried thyme, dried rosemary, and minced garlic. Brush each lamb chop with a thin layer of Dijon mustard. This will help the herb crust adhere.

Press the breadcrumb mixture firmly onto both sides of the lamb chops, ensuring they are evenly coated. In an oven-safe skillet, heat the olive oil over medium-high heat. Once the oil is hot, add the lamb chops and sear them on each side (about a couple of minutes per side but if the meat is cut thickly 3 minutes) until they form a lightly browned crust.

Once the lamb chops are cooked to your liking, remove the pan from the oven and let the chops rest for a few minutes. This resting period allows the juices to redistribute throughout the meat, ensuring a tender and flavorful result. Serve the lamb chops hot and enjoy their rich, savory taste.

Nutrition: | Calories: 301 | Fat: 14 g | Carbs: 9 g | Sugar: 4 g | Protein: 27 g

Chicken and Peppers

Prep Time
5 min

Cook Time
20 min

Servings
2

Ingredients
2 boneless, skinless chicken breasts
salt to taste
2 tablespoons extra virgin olive oil
1 red bell pepper and 1 yellow bell pepper, thinly sliced
1 onion, thinly sliced
2 cloves garlic, minced
1/2 teaspoon dried oregano and paprika
1/2 teaspoon dried basil
Fresh parsley, chopped (for garnish)
Lemon wedges (for serving)

Preparation

Season the chicken breasts generously with salt on both sides.

In a large skillet over medium-high heat, heat the extra-virgin olive oil.

Carefully place the chicken breasts in the skillet and cook for about 5-7 minutes per side, (depending on the thickness of the chicken slices).

Next, remove the chicken breasts from the skillet and set aside to rest.

In the same skillet, add the sliced peppers and onion and sauté for about 5 minutes, stirring occasionally, until they become tender and begin to caramelize. The remaining flavors of the chicken will enhance the taste of the peppers and onions.

Continue cooking until the vegetables are softened. Return the cooked chicken breasts to the skillet, placing them among the peppers and onions.

Reduce the heat to medium-low and allow the chicken and peppers to simmer together for another 5 minutes to meld the flavors.

Garnish with chopped fresh parsley and serve the pan-seared chicken and peppers hot, accompanied by lemon wedges for squeezing over the dish.

Nutrition |Calories: 196 | Fat:9 g |Carbs: 1 g |Sugar: 0 g |Protein: 29 g

Turkey with Pumpkin Curry

Prep Time
10 min

Cook Time
20 min

Servings
2

Ingredients

200g lean ground turkey (93% lean or higher)

1 cup pumpkin puree (unsweetened)

1/2 cup coconut milk

2 garlic cloves, minced

1 small onion, finely chopped

1-inch piece of fresh ginger, grated

1 tbsp curry powder

1/2 tsp ground turmeric

1/4 tsp ground cumin and cinnamon

1 tbsp extra virgin olive oil

Salt and pepper to taste

Fresh cilantro for garnish (optional)

For Serving:

1/2 cup cooked brown rice or quinoa (optional, for extra fiber)

Steamed vegetables (e.g., spinach, green beans, or broccoli)

Preparation

Heat olive oil in a large skillet over medium heat and cook the ground turkey for 5-7 minutes until browned. Season with salt and pepper, then set aside.

In the same skillet, sauté garlic, onion and ginger for 2-3 minutes until fragrant.

Add curry powder, turmeric, cumin, and cinnamon, cooking for another minute. Stir in pumpkin puree and coconut milk, simmer for 5-7 minutes.

Return the turkey to the skillet, mix, and simmer for an additional 3-5 minutes. Adjust seasoning to taste.

Serve: Divide the turkey pumpkin curry between two plates. Garnish with fresh cilantro if desired and serve with a side of brown rice or quinoa and steamed vegetables.

Nutrition | Calories: 310 | Fat: 21 g | Carbs: 14 g | Sugar: 0 g | Protein: 29 g

FISH BASED DISHES

Lemon Herb Salmon

Prep Time

5 min

Cook Time

15 min

Servings

2

Ingredients
2 salmon fillets

Salt and pepper to taste

2 tablespoons olive oil

2 cloves garlic, minced

1 lemon, sliced

1 tablespoon fresh parsley, chopped

1 tablespoon fresh dill, chopped

1 tablespoon fresh chives, chopped

Preparation
Preheat your oven to 400°F (200°C).

In a small bowl, combine the oil, garlic, herbs, and lemon juice. Line a baking dish with parchment paper and place the salmon fillets inside. Brush the oil mixture evenly over each fillet, ensuring they are well coated.

Finally, add salt garnish each fillet with a few thin lemon slices Transfer the pan to the oven and bake the fillets for about 12 to 15 minutes.

Once cooked, serve the salmon with an additional drizzle of raw extra-virgin olive oil and fresh lemon wedges on the side for extra flavor.

Enjoy this delicious and aromatic dish!

Nutrition: |Calories: 302 | Fat: 24 g |Carbs: 2 g |Sugar: 0 g |Protein: 24 g

Garlic Herb Fish Skewers

Prep Time
10 min

Cook Time
15 min

Servings
2

Ingredients

8 large shrimp, peeled and deveined

8 sea scallops

1/4 cup olive oil

2 cloves garlic, minced

a pinch of dried thyme

2 tbsp lemon juice

1 tsp dried oregano

a pinch of salt and black pepper

2 skewers

Preparation

Preheat your grill or grill pan over medium-high heat.

Prepare Marinade: In a small bowl, combine minced garlic, olive oil, chopped parsley, chopped dill, salt, and pepper. Mix well to create the marinade.

Thread the fish chunks and lemon slices onto the soaked wooden skewers, alternating between fish and lemon.

Brush the garlic herb marinade generously over the fish skewers, ensuring they are well coated on all sides.

Position the skewers onto the heated grill or grill pan and cook for 4-5 minutes on each side.

Once cooked, remove the fish skewers from the grill and serve hot with additional lemon wedges and fresh herbs on the side.

Nutrition: |Calories: 298 | Fat: 16 g | Carbs: 4 g | Sugar: 0 g | Protein: 20 g

Salmon with Honey Glaze

Prep Time

5 min

Cook Time

10 min

Servings

2

Ingredients
2 salmon fillets

2 tablespoons honey

1 tablespoon soy sauce

1 tablespoon canola oil

1 teaspoon minced garlic and ginger

salt and pepper to taste

Sesame seeds for garnish

sliced green onions for garnish

Preparation

Combine the honey, soy sauce, minced garlic, and grated ginger in a bowl to create the glaze.

In a large skillet over medium-high heat, warm the canola oil and once hot, add the seasoned salmon fillets to the skillet, placing them skin-side down. Add salt and pepper. Cook for 3-4 minutes until the skin becomes crispy and golden brown.

Add Glaze: Carefully flip the salmon fillets using a spatula. Pour the honey glaze over the fillets, allowing it to coat the salmon evenly.

Continue to cook the salmon for an additional 3-4 minutes, basting the fillets with the glaze occasionally, until the salmon is cooked through and flakes easily with a fork.

Serve: Transfer the fillets to serving plates. For an added touch of flavor and visual appeal, sprinkle the salmon with sesame seeds and sliced green onions. Serve the hot, flavorful salmon with your choice of side dishes, such as steamed vegetables or whole grain rice, to create a balanced and satisfying meal.

Nutrition: |Calories: 213 | Fat: 10 g |Carbs: 3 g |Sugar: 1 g |Protein: 28 g

Cod with Roasted Tomato

Prep Time
5 min

Cook Time
10 min

Servings
2

Ingredients

2 cod fillets

2 cups cherry tomatoes

3 cloves garlic, minced

2 tablespoons canola oil

1 teaspoon dried oregano

1 teaspoon dried basil

Salt and pepper to taste

Fresh parsley for garnish

Preparation

Preheat the oven to 400°F (200°C).

Arrange the cherry tomatoes on a parchment-lined baking sheet. Drizzle them with canola oil and sprinkle with minced garlic, dried oregano, dried basil, salt, and pepper. Toss the tomatoes to ensure even coating.

Roast the cherry tomatoes in the preheated oven for 15-20.

Season both sides of the cod fillets with salt and pepper.

In a large skillet over medium heat, heat the remaining canola oil. Add the seasoned cod fillets to the skillet and cook for 3-4 minutes on each side until the fish is fully cooked and easily flakes with a fork.

Remove the cherry from the oven and gently mash them with a fork to release more juices and divide the roasted cherry tomato sauce between two plates and place a cooked cod fillet on each portion.

Garnish with fresh parsley and serve hot.

Nutrition: | Calories: 213 | Fat: 10 g | Carbs: 3 g | Sugar: 1 g | Protein: 28 g

Salmon with Avocado and Feta Crumble

Prep Time	Cook Time	Servings
5 min	15 min	2

Ingredients

2 salmon fillets

1 ripe avocado, diced

1/4 cup crumbled feta cheese

1 tbsp lemon juice and 2 tbsp extra virgin olive oil

2 cloves garlic, minced

Salt and pepper to taste

Fresh parsley for garnish

Preparation

Preheat the oven to 400°F (200°C).

Season the salmon fillets with salt, pepper, and minced garlic.

Drizzle 1 tablespoon of olive oil and lemon juice over the seasoned salmon fillets.

Place the seasoned salmon fillets on a baking sheet lined with parchment paper, ensuring they are spaced out evenly for proper cooking. Transfer the baking sheet to the preheated oven and bake the fillets for 12-15 minutes.

Monitor the salmon closely until it is fully cooked and flakes effortlessly with a fork, indicating it has reached the perfect level of doneness. The gentle baking process will ensure the salmon remains moist and flavorful..

Prepare Avocado and Feta Crumble: In a small bowl, combine the diced avocado and crumbled feta cheese. Season with salt and pepper to taste.

Gently mash the avocado and feta together with a fork until well combined but still chunky.

Serve: Once the salmon is done baking, remove it from the oven and transfer it to serving plates. Top each salmon fillet with the avocado and feta crumble.
Garnish: Garnish with fresh parsley leaves for an extra pop of color and flavor.

Nutrition: |Calories: 260 | Fat: 10 g |Carbs: 24 g |Protein: 26 g

Cod in Parsley Cream Sauce

Prep Time
10 min

Cook Time
15 min

Servings
2

Ingredients
2 cod fillets
1 tbsp avocado oil
1/2 cup unsweetened almond milk
1 tbsp whole wheat flour
1/4 cup vegetable broth (preferably organic)
1/4 cup fresh parsley, finely chopped
1 clove garlic, minced
1 tbsp lemon juice
alt and pepper to taste
Lemon wedges (optional)
For Serving:
Steamed or roasted vegetables (e.g., broccoli, carrots, zucchini)
Quinoa or brown rice (optional, for extra fiber)

Preparation

Cook the cod: Heat 1/2 tablespoon of avocado oil in a non-stick pan over medium heat. Season the cod with salt and pepper, then cook for 3-4 minutes per side until it flakes easily. Remove and set aside.

For the parsley cream sauce: In the same pan, add the remaining avocado oil and garlic. Sauté for 1 minute until fragrant.

Make the sauce base: Sprinkle the flour over the garlic and stir to combine, cooking for 1 minute. Slowly whisk in the almond milk and vegetable broth, making sure the sauce is smooth and lump-free. Simmer for 2-3 minutes, letting the sauce thicken slightly as the flavors blend. Stir occasionally to prevent sticking. Add parsley and lemon: Stir in the chopped parsley and lemon juice, and season with salt and pepper to taste. Cook for another 1-2 minutes until the sauce is fragrant and well-blended.

Finish and serve: Return the cooked cod to the skillet, spooning some of the parsley cream sauce over the top. Simmer for another 2-3 minutes to heat through and allow the flavors to meld.

Serve: Plate the cod fillets, drizzling the parsley cream sauce over them. Serve with steamed or roasted vegetables and a side of quinoa or brown rice if desired. Top off the dish with lemon wedges for a bright, fresh touch.

Nutrition: |Calories: 245 | Fat: 9 g |Carbs: 7 g |Sugar: 1 g |Protein: 30 g

LOW SUGAR

DESSERTS

Almond Flour Chocolate Cake

Prep Time
10 min

Cook Time
10 min

Servings
10

Dry Ingredients:
1/2 cup unsweetened cocoa powder
1/2 cup granulated erythritol (low-carb sweetener)
2 cups almond flour
1 tsp baking powder
A pinch of salt

Wet Ingredients:
3 large eggs
1/2 cup unsweetened almond milk
1/2 cup melted coconut oil or unsalted butter
1 tsp vanilla extract

Preparation

Preheat the oven to 175°C (350°F).

Line a round cake pan (8 inch) with parchment paper.

Mix Dry Ingredients: In a large bowl, mix together all the dry ingredients, excluding the erythritol, until well combined.

Mix Wet Ingredients: In another bowl, beat the eggs with the erythritol until slightly frothy.

Add the melted coconut oil (or butter), almond milk, and vanilla extract, and mix until you get a smooth mixture.

Pour the wet ingredients into the bowl with the dry ingredients and gently mix until just combined.

If desired, fold in the sugar-free dark chocolate chips or chopped nuts.

Pour the batter into the prepared cake pan, leveling the surface.

Bake for 28-30 minutes, or until a toothpick inserted into the center comes out clean.

Let the cake cool in the pan for 10 minutes, then transfer to a wire rack to cool completely.

Optionally, you can dust it with cocoa powder.

Nutrition: |Calories: 339 | Fat: 28 g |Carbs: 6 g |Sugar: 5 g |Protein: 14 g

Vanilla Brownies

Prep Time
10 min

Cook Time
25 min

Servings
12

Dry Ingredients:
1 1/2 cups almond flour
1/2 cup granulated erythritol (low-carb sweetener)
1/4 cup coconut flour
1 tsp baking powder
1/4 tsp salt

Wet Ingredients:
4 large eggs, at room temperature
1/2 cup unsweetened almond milk
1/2 cup melted coconut oil or unsalted butter
2 tsp vanilla extract
Optional Add-Ins:
1/2 cup sugar-free white chocolate chips
1/4 cup chopped pecans or walnuts

Preparation

Preheat the oven to 175°C (350°F) and prepare a baking pan (8x8 inch) by lining it with parchment paper.

Mix Dry Ingredients: In a large bowl, combine the almond flour, coconut flour, baking powder, and salt.

Mix Wet Ingredients: In a separate bowl, beat the eggs with the erythritol until slightly frothy.

Add the melted coconut oil (or butter), almond milk, and vanilla extract to the eggs, whisking until you achieve a smooth consistency.

Pour the wet ingredients into the bowl with the dry ingredients and gently mix until just combined.

If desired, fold in the sugar-free white chocolate chips and chopped nuts.

Pour the batter into the prepared baking pan, spreading it evenly with a spatula.

Bake the Brownies: Place the pan in the oven and bake for 20-25 minutes, until the surface is golden and slightly firm to the touch.

Cool and Serve:

Let the brownies cool in the pan for a minimum of 10 minutes,

Once cooled, cut the brownies into slices.

Nutrition: |Calories: 324 | Fat: 18 g |Carbs: 9 g |Sugar: 4 g |Protein: 12 g

Baked Apples with Cinnamon and Walnuts

Prep Time
5 min

Cook Time
10 min

Servings
2

Ingredients

2 medium apples (e.g., Granny Smith, Honeycrisp, or Fuji)

2 tbsp chopped walnuts

1 tbsp ground flaxseed (optional, for added fiber)

1 tsp ground cinnamon

1/2 tsp vanilla extract

1 tsp pure maple syrup (optional, or use stevia for no added sugar)

1/4 cup unsweetened almond milk

extra virgin olive oil for greasing

For Serving:

2 tbsp plain, unsweetened Greek yogurt or dairy-free yogurt (optional)

Preparation

Prepare the apples: Preheat the oven to 350°F (175°C). Use an apple corer or paring knife to remove the core while keeping the base intact, creating a hollow space for the filling.

Make the filling: In a small bowl, mix the chopped walnuts, flaxseed (if using), cinnamon, maple syrup (or stevia), and vanilla extract.

Stuff the apples: Place the apples in a small baking dish and fill each apple cavity with the walnut mixture. Pour the almond milk around the apples in the dish to keep them moist while baking.

Bake the apples: Lightly spray the tops of the apples with a tiny amount of olive oil. Bake the apples for 20-25 minutes, or until they are soft and the filling turns golden brown. You can cover them with aluminum foil midway through to prevent excessive browning if necessary.

Serve: Let the baked apples cool slightly. Serve warm with a spoonful of unsweetened Greek yogurt or dairy-free yogurt on top for added creaminess if desired.

Nutrition: |Calories: 175 | Fat: 8 g |Carbs: 23 g |Sugar: 4 g |Protein: 4 g

Comprehensive 28-Day Meal Plan

DAY	BREAKFAST	LUNCH	DINNER	SNACK
1	Cottage Cheese Pancakes with Coffee	Quinoa Salad with Raw Carrot Sticks	Savory Herb-Crusted Beef with Baked Brussels Sprouts	Almonds with Fresh Berries of Your Choice
2	Green Omelette with Green Tea	Lentil Croquettes with Raw Cucumber Slices	Lemon Herb Salmon with Roasted Broccoli	Walnuts and Olives
3	Avocado and Egg Bowl with Ginger Herbal Tea	Chickpea Salad with Raw Bell Pepper Strips	Grilled Meats with Tzatziki Sauce and Baked Sweet Potato	Walnuts with Fresh Berries of Your Choice
4	Egg-cellent Chicken Bites with Coffee	Quinoa Bowl with Cooked Spinach	Super Chicken Tenders with Raw Celery Sticks	Sugar-Free Yogurt with Blueberries
5	Italian Style Eggs with Green Tea	Veggie Stir-Fry with Cooked Zucchini	Steak Bites and Mushrooms with Baked Brussels Sprouts	Celery or Fennel with Brazil Nuts
6	Blueberry Flan with Ginger Herbal Tea	Quinoa Salad with Raw Carrot Sticks	Mediterranean Veal Medallions with Roasted Cauliflower	Walnuts and Olives

7	Mini Cinnamon Biscuits with Coffee	Lentil Croquettes with Cooked Spinach	Herb-Crusted Lamb Chops with Baked Sweet Potato	Walnuts and Olives
8	Zucchini Pie with Green Tea	Chickpea Salad with Raw Bell Pepper Strips	Super Crispy Chicken Wings with Cooked Broccoli	Sugar-Free Yogurt with Raspberries
9	Breakfast Pizza with Ginger Herbal Tea	Quinoa Bowl with Raw Cucumber Slices	Lemon Herb Salmon with Cooked Brussels Sprouts	Walnuts with Fresh Berries of Your Choice
10	Cottage Cheese Pancakes with Coffee	Veggie Stir-Fry with Raw Celery Sticks	Grilled Meats with Tzatziki Sauce and Baked Sweet Potato	Walnuts and Olives
11	Green Omelette with Green Tea	Chickpea Salad with Cooked Spinach	Steak Bites and Mushrooms with Raw Carrot Sticks	Celery or Fennel with Brazil Nuts
12	Avocado and Egg Bowl with Ginger Herbal Tea	Quinoa Salad with Raw Bell Pepper Strips	Herb-Crusted Lamb Chops with Baked Brussels Sprouts	Sugar-Free Yogurt with Blackberries
13	Egg-cellent Chicken Bites with Coffee	Lentil Croquettes with Cooked Zucchini	Mediterranean Veal Medallions with Raw Cucumber Slices	Celery or Fennel with Brazil Nuts

14	Italian Style Eggs with Green Tea	Quinoa Bowl with Raw Celery Sticks	Super Chicken Tenders with Cooked Broccoli	Walnuts with Fresh Berries of Your Choice
15	Blueberry Flan with Ginger Herbal Tea	Chickpea Salad with Cooked Spinach	Lemon Herb Salmon with Baked Sweet Potato	Celery or Fennel with Brazil Nuts
16	Mini Cinnamon Biscuits with Coffee	Quinoa Salad with Raw Carrot Sticks	Steak Bites and Mushrooms with Raw Bell Pepper Strips	Sugar-Free Yogurt with Blueberries
17	Zucchini Pie with Green Tea	Lentil Croquettes with Raw Cucumber Slices	Herb-Crusted Lamb Chops with Baked Brussels Sprouts	Walnuts with Fresh Berries of Your Choice
18	Cottage Cheese Pancakes with Ginger Herbal Tea	Veggie Stir-Fry with Cooked Zucchini	Grilled Meats with Tzatziki Sauce and Raw Carrot Sticks	Celery or Fennel with Brazil Nuts
19	Green Omelette with Coffee	Chickpea Salad with Raw Bell Pepper Strips	Lemon Herb Salmon with Cooked Brussels Sprouts	Sugar-Free Yogurt with Raspberries
20	Avocado and Egg Bowl with Green Tea	Quinoa Salad with Raw Cucumber Slices	Mediterranean Veal Medallions with Baked Sweet Potato	Walnuts with Fresh Berries of Your Choice

21	Egg-cellent Chicken Bites with Ginger Herbal Tea	Veggie Stir-Fry with Raw Carrot Sticks	Super Chicken Tenders with Cooked Broccoli	Olives
22	Italian Style Eggs with Coffee	Lentil Croquettes with Cooked Zucchini	Steak Bites and Mushrooms with Raw Bell Pepper Strips	Almonds with Fresh Berries of Your Choice
23	Blueberry Flan with Green Tea	Chickpea Salad with Cooked Spinach	Herb-Crusted Lamb Chops with Baked Brussels Sprouts	Sugar-Free Yogurt with Blackberries
24	Mini Cinnamon Biscuits with Ginger Herbal Tea	Quinoa Bowl with Raw Cucumber Slices	Grilled Meats with Tzatziki Sauce and Baked Sweet Potato	Olives
25	Zucchini Pie with Coffee	Lentil Croquettes with Raw Carrot Sticks	Mediterranean Veal Medallions with Cooked Spinach	Dried Figs
26	Cottage Cheese Pancakes with Green Tea	Quinoa Salad with Raw Bell Pepper Strips	Super Chicken Tenders with Baked Brussels Sprouts	Celery or Fennel with Brazil Nuts
27	Green Omelette with Ginger Herbal Tea	Chickpea Salad with Cooked Spinach	Lemon Herb Salmon with Raw Cucumber Slices	Sugar-Free Yogurt with Raspberries

28	Avocado and Egg Bowl with Coffee	Veggie Stir-Fry with Raw Bell Pepper Strips	Herb-Crusted Lamb Chops with Baked Sweet Potato	Walnuts with Fresh Berries of Your Choice

DOWNLOAD HERE YOUR FREE BONUS

5 Best Tips to Revers Fatty Liver

Is it true that coffee consumption can have positive effects on fatty liver disease?

The optimal exercise program for those aiming to reverse fatty liver

10 Delicious Detox Smoothie Recipes

Best supplements for fatty liver

Written by Dr. Maggie A. Whit

1